# Simplified Solution Approach

# To **SICKLE CELL ANEMIA**

Unlocking the Path to Vitality: A Comprehensive Guide to Overcoming the Chains of Genetic Challenges

# Dr QUENTIN GLYN

# Table Of Contents

# CHAPTER ONE
## Sickle Cell Anemia

The inherited blood condition known as sickle cell anemia (SCA) is characterized by aberrant hemoglobin in red blood cells called hemoglobin S (HbS). Red blood cells with this disorder have a sickle or crescent form, which may result in a number of problems including discomfort, anemia, and organ damage. Certain groups are more likely to have sickle cell anemia than others, especially individuals of African, Mediterranean, Middle Eastern, and Indian heritage.

## Sickle Cell Anemia Overview:

Investigating Sickle Cell Anemia at the molecular level is crucial to comprehending its effects. The mutation that causes HbS to arise occurs in hemoglobin, the protein that carries oxygen in the blood. Red blood cells may become sticky and stiff due to these aberrant hemoglobin molecules under some situations, which can clog tiny blood arteries. Pain, tissue damage, and reduced blood supply to different organs may arise from this.

Sickle cell anemia may cause modest to severe clinical symptoms, such as recurring bouts of discomfort, exhaustion, and an increased risk of infections. Nearly every organ system is susceptible to complications, including the brain, kidneys, lungs, and spleen. The disease's chronic nature significantly impairs the quality of life for affected people and their families.

## The Need To Treat Sickle Cell Anemia:

Sickle cell anemia has a significant worldwide effect, especially in areas where it is very prevalent. The illness has a significant financial impact on communities and healthcare systems in addition to having a physical impact on patients. Furthermore, it is important to recognize the psychological effects of having a chronic disease since these individuals often experience stigma and have difficulty getting access to quality treatment and support.

The treatment of sickle cell anemia goes beyond the disease's acute symptoms. It entails a thorough strategy that includes targeted therapy development, early identification, genetic counseling, and problem management. It is impossible to overestimate the significance of advancing research, creating a supportive atmosphere, and increasing awareness for people with SCA.

## The Book's Goal: A Simplified Approach To Solving Problems:

The goal of this book is to provide clear and thorough guidance for understanding and managing sickle cell anemia. While acknowledging the condition's complexity, it makes an effort to simplify the material so that patients, caregivers, medical professionals, and the general public can all understand it.

This book's streamlined solution method highlights the need for a multifaceted approach. It includes early screening, lifestyle modifications to control symptoms, and genetic risk factor education. The book also looks at new developments in medical research and treatment alternatives, which may lead to discoveries that provide hope for those with sickle cell anemia.

This book seeks to educate readers on Sickle Cell Anemia from a holistic standpoint, debunk common misconceptions about the illness, and build a supportive community among its readers.

The aim is to improve the lives of individuals impacted by this difficult genetic illness by lowering stigma, increasing knowledge, and eventually improving SCA via a streamlined solution approach.

# CHAPTER TWO

## Knowledge About Anemia Sickle Cell

Red blood cells with sickle cell anemia have an unusual form, which is indicative of a hereditary condition. Red blood cells in a healthy person are round, flexible, and disc-shaped, which makes it easy for them to pass through blood channels and provide oxygen to different parts of the body. However, a genetic mutation that results in the creation of aberrant hemoglobin, called hemoglobin S, causes sickle cell anemia.

Red blood cells with this changed hemoglobin become stiff and resemble a crescent or sickle shapes.

A genetic mutation in the HBB gene, which codes for the production of hemoglobin's beta-globin component, is the main cause of sickle cell anemia. Instead of the typical hemoglobin A, hemoglobin S is produced as a result of this mutation. For the disease to appear, an individual must inherit the mutant gene from both parents.

## Genetic Foundation And Heredity

Sickle cell anemia is inherited in an autosomal recessive manner. This indicates that in order to have the condition, a person has to inherit two copies of the defective gene, one from each parent.

A person is referred to be a carrier or heterozygote if they inherit one copy of the mutant gene and one copy of the normal gene. Despite being asymptomatic carriers, heterozygotes have the ability to pass on the defective gene to their progeny.

In areas where malaria is or was endemic, the HBB gene mutation that causes sickle cell anemia is more common. This is due to the fact that people who are heterozygotes—those who only have one copy of the defective gene—show greater resistance to malaria. As a result, the prevalence of the sickle cell gene in the population is greater in regions where malaria is prevalent.

# The Signs And Symptoms

Sickle cell anemia symptoms may vary greatly from person to person and can also evolve over time. The defining characteristic is the red blood cell sickling, which may result in a number of problems. Typical signs and symptoms include:

Agony Crises: Periods of extreme agony are called pain crises because sickle-shaped red blood cells might obstruct blood flow. These crises might vary in length and intensity and impact various bodily areas.

Anemia: Chronic low red blood cell count, or anemia, is caused by sickle cells, which have shorter lives than healthy red blood cells. Weakness, exhaustion, and pale complexion may all be signs of anemia.

Organ Damage: Recurrent instances of blood flow obstruction may cause harm to tissues and organs. The liver, kidneys, and spleen are often impacted, which may result in a number of issues.

Infections: Because of the impaired function of the spleen, individuals with sickle cell anemia are more vulnerable to infections. The removal of microorganisms from the bloodstream is a critical function of the spleen.

Jaundice: The disintegration of sickle cells may produce bilirubin, which causes the skin and eyes to become yellow.

Delayed Growth: The long-term impact of sickle cell anemia on the body might cause delays in a child's growth and development.

In summary, knowledge of sickle cell anemia requires an awareness of its genetic foundation, pattern of inheritance, and range of symptoms and manifestations. In addition to affecting the structure and functionality of red blood cells, this genetic condition has systemic repercussions that may have a major negative influence on a person's health and quality of life.

# CHAPTER THREE

## Identification And Prompt Diagnosis

### Methods For Screening And Diagnosis:

A genetic blood condition known as sickle cell anemia (SCA) is characterized by the presence of hemoglobin S, an aberrant form of hemoglobin.

Early diagnosis and detection of sickle cell anemia are essential for successful treatment of the illness. Different screening and diagnostic techniques are essential for identifying people with SCA.

Newborn screening, which is done soon after delivery, is one of the main screening techniques. This is a straightforward blood test to identify any aberrant hemoglobin levels. Programs for newborn screening have shown to be quite successful in detecting babies with SCA, enabling management and early intervention.

Hemoglobin electrophoresis and high-performance liquid chromatography (HPLC) are two laboratory procedures used to diagnose sickle cell anemia. By distinguishing between hemoglobin S and normal hemoglobin, these methods aid in making a conclusive diagnosis. Another effective method is genetic testing, which makes it possible to pinpoint certain genetic mutations linked to SCA.

# The Value Of Early Identification:

For a number of reasons, early identification of sickle cell anemia is essential. First of all, it makes it easier to intervene early and start proper medical therapy, both of which may greatly enhance the quality of life for those who have the illness. Prompt diagnosis further facilitates early illness education for patients and their families, empowering them to make knowledgeable choices about available treatments and lifestyle modifications.

Moreover, problems from sickle cell anemia must be avoided with early identification. Prophylactic interventions, such as immunization and antibiotic medication, may be started on time to help lower the risk of infections, which are major consequences in people with SCA. It becomes feasible to conduct routine monitoring and medical follow-ups, guaranteeing that any new health problems are dealt with right away.

## Problems With Diagnosis:

Even though early diagnosis is crucial, identifying sickle cell anemia may be difficult for a number of reasons. One problem is that the disorder might be hard to diagnose based alone on clinical presentation due to the wide range of symptoms, from moderate to severe. Underdiagnosis might result from this diversity, particularly in situations with less severe symptoms.

Lack of access to healthcare resources may also make it difficult to conduct screening programs that are successful, especially in low-income areas. Delayed diagnosis may also result from a lack of understanding about the significance of early detection among the general public and healthcare professionals.

Sickle cell anemia diagnosis depends on genetic counseling, yet there are obstacles to overcome, including cultural stigmas, fear, and misunderstandings about genetic testing. A comprehensive strategy including community involvement, education, and the creation of an infrastructure for accessible healthcare is needed to overcome these obstacles.

In conclusion, a mix of screening and diagnostic techniques is used in the diagnosis and early identification of sickle cell anemia. For better patient outcomes, proper therapy, and the avoidance of problems, early diagnosis is essential. However, in order to guarantee that people with SCA get early and appropriate treatment, diagnostic problems such as symptom unpredictability and restricted access to healthcare facilities must be addressed.

# CHAPTER FOUR

# Present Therapies And Their Restrictions

**Synopsis Of Current Therapies:**
A hereditary condition known as sickle cell anemia (SCA) is characterized by aberrant hemoglobin, which gives red blood cells a stiff, sickle-like form. The goals of the current SCA therapies are to reduce symptoms, control complications, and enhance the general well-being of those who are impacted. The following strategies are used in the management of SCA:

1. Pain management is a crucial component of therapy for SCA patients since pain is one of the disease's primary symptoms. Pain

management practitioners often prescribe analgesic medicines, such as opioids and nonsteroidal anti-inflammatory drugs (NSAIDs), to treat both acute and chronic pain.

2. Hydroxyurea Therapy: Studies have shown that Hydroxyurea increases fetal hemoglobin synthesis, improving red blood cell deformability and lowering the frequency of excruciating crises.

3. Blood Transfusions: Red blood cell transfusions are used to treat severe anemia and boost the blood's ability to transport oxygen. On the other hand, iron overload brought on by repeated transfusions may need further chelation therapy treatment to eliminate extra iron.

4. Bone Marrow Transplantation: This possibly curative approach for sickle cell anemia (SCA) involves using a suitable donor's bone marrow in lieu of the patient's own. The danger of problems and the availability of appropriate donors, however, restrict the approach's broad use.

## Constraints And Adverse Reactions:

Although these therapies provide some alleviation, they have drawbacks and possible adverse consequences.

1. Painkillers: NSAIDs may result in stomach problems, and long-term usage of opioids may create dependency and addiction. Furthermore, severe pain episodes

cannot always be prevented or lessened by pain treatment.

2. Hydroxyurea: Myelosuppression, or decreased formation of blood cells, gastrointestinal issues, and skin responses are possible adverse effects for some people. The long-term safety of it is still being looked at.

3. Blood Transfusions: Iron excess brought on by repeated transfusions may cause problems including damage to organs, particularly the liver and heart. Although chelation treatment works well, it comes with a lot of drawbacks.

4. Bone Marrow Transplantation: This surgery has a number of substantial hazards, such as death from transplant-related causes

and graft-versus-host disease. It may be difficult to find acceptable donors, and not everyone is a good fit for this strategy.

## Views From Patients:

It is essential to comprehend the viewpoints and experiences of people with SCA in order to customize therapies to meet their requirements. Patients often voice worries about managing their medicines, the unpredictable nature of their condition, and the effect of chronic pain on their everyday lives. The shortcomings of existing therapies highlight the need for further investigation and the creation of fresh therapeutic strategies that deal with the underlying causes of SCA.

In conclusion, while some alleviation from SCA is offered by existing therapies, these interventions have drawbacks and may cause adverse reactions. In order to create more efficient and user-friendly medicines for the management of sickle cell anemia, patient viewpoints are crucial.

# CHAPTER FIVE

## Prospective Studies And Innovations

### Progress In Gene Therapy:

Gene therapy has significant potential in the management of hereditary illnesses like sickle cell anemia. This method addresses the underlying cause of the illness by adjusting or changing the patient's DNA.

Researchers have made great progress in creating gene treatments for sickle cell anemia, which attempt to fix the genetic abnormalities causing aberrant hemoglobin synthesis.

One significant development is the use of CRISPR-Cas9 technology, a ground-breaking gene-editing instrument that enables researchers to precisely alter the DNA sequence. Scientists have been investigating how to modify the genes that produce hemoglobin using CRISPR-Cas9 in order to fix the defect linked to sickle cell anemia. Promising findings from preclinical studies and early research have raised expectations for a possible curative therapy.

## Creative Methods Of Treatment:

In addition to gene therapy, several therapeutic modalities have been developed with the goal of better controlling sickle cell anemia and raising the standard of living for affected individuals. Fetal hemoglobin inducers are one method of doing this. Compared to hemoglobin normally present in adults, fetal hemoglobin, which is created during fetal development, has a greater ability to transport oxygen.

Researchers have been looking at substances and medications that might help people with sickle cell anemia produce more fetal hemoglobin. It is feasible to lessen the consequences of the disease's aberrant hemoglobin by raising fetal hemoglobin levels, which will reduce sickle cell crises and problems.

## Clinical Trials: Overview And Outcomes:

Clinical trials are often used to conduct rigorous testing in order to translate promising research into effective medicines.

A large number of clinical studies have been carried out to assess the effectiveness and safety of new treatments for sickle cell anemia. A wide range of individuals, including those with various genotypes and illness severity, usually participate in these studies.

A few studies evaluate the safety and long-term impacts of gene-editing technologies with an emphasis on gene therapy treatments. Others investigate the effectiveness of cutting-edge medications and therapeutic modalities, such as new anti-sickling agents or fetal hemoglobin inducers. The outcomes of these clinical trials direct researchers to hone their techniques and provide vital insights into the possibilities of these medicines.

All things considered, the field of sickle cell anemia research is changing quickly thanks to exciting developments in gene therapy, creative therapeutic strategies, and positive outcomes from clinical trials. Even if there are still obstacles to overcome, these developments provide people with sickle cell anemia hope for a better future by presenting the prospect of more powerful and maybe even curative therapies.

# CHAPTER SIX

## Changes In Lifestyle And Holistic Care

Managing sickle cell anemia holistically addresses the physical, emotional, and social aspects of the patient in addition to standard medical therapies. This strategy seeks to improve the general quality of life for people with sickle cell anemia by acknowledging the interdependence of several variables impacting health and well-being.

## The Significance Of A Holistic Approach:

1. Wholesome Well-Being: A holistic approach takes the patient's condition into

account, realizing that mental and emotional health are closely related to physical health. This method acknowledges that providing treatment for symptoms alone may not be enough and that complete care requires addressing the underlying causes and contributing factors.

2. Patient Empowerment: People with sickle cell anemia who get holistic treatment are able to take an active role in managing their health. This includes telling patients about their illnesses, supporting self-care routines, and giving them a feeling of control over their well-being.

3. Long-term Benefits: A comprehensive approach might possibly lessen the frequency and intensity of sickle cell crises

by addressing lifestyle variables and mental well-being. By providing a supportive atmosphere for the patient, it may also increase the efficacy of medical therapies.

## Dietary Advice:

1. Balanced Diet: People with sickle cell anemia must eat a diet rich in nutrients. To encourage the creation of healthy red blood cells and avoid difficulties, it's critical to consume an adequate amount of minerals including iron, folic acid, and vitamin B12.

2. Water: People with sickle cell anemia must maintain enough water since dehydration may worsen symptoms and raise the possibility of crises. Maintaining enough hydration lowers the viscosity of

sickle-shaped red blood cells and aids in blood flow maintenance.

3. Supplementation: To treat certain deficits, it may sometimes be advised to take nutritional supplements. For example, folic acid supplements may help control the symptoms of anemia and encourage the synthesis of red blood cells.

## Changes In Lifestyle To Enhance Quality Of Life:

1. Frequent Exercise: Moderate to vigorous physical activity should be avoided while dealing with sickle cell crises, although frequent exercise may improve general health. Engaging in physical exercise

promotes stress reduction, better circulation, and healthy weight maintenance.

2. Stress management: Sickle cell crises may be brought on by prolonged stress. Methods like yoga, meditation, and deep breathing may help lower stress levels, increase relaxation, and lessen the chance of problems.

3. Sleep hygiene: Those who have sickle cell anemia must get enough rest. Regular sleep schedules and suitable sleeping environments may help improve general health and lower the risk of consequences from exhaustion.

4. Social Support: For those who are dealing with a chronic illness, developing a solid support system is essential. Developing a

feeling of community and receiving emotional support might come from interacting with others who are aware of the difficulties associated with sickle cell anemia.

In summary, dietary counseling and lifestyle changes are essential components of a comprehensive therapy strategy for sickle cell anemia patients. This method aims to promote total well-being and enable patients to lead satisfying lives despite the obstacles given by the disease by addressing the physical, emotional, and social components of the person.

# CHAPTER SEVEN

## Patient Support And Empowerment

A comprehensive strategy that extends beyond pharmaceutical interventions is needed to treat sickle cell anemia. It is essential to empower people in order to improve their general health.

This entails giving them a feeling of agency and control over how they manage their illness. In order to enable patients to actively participate in their own health, support from medical professionals, families, and the community is essential.

# Advocacy And Patient Education:

Effective therapy for sickle cell anemia requires educating patients about the condition. Information on the disease's nature, possible treatments, and lifestyle modifications are all included in this. Education and advocacy go hand in hand since they both include raising public knowledge of sickle cell anemia. This may result in better support networks, less stigma, and more understanding for people who are impacted by the illness.

## Resources And Support Systems:

Establishing and maintaining support systems is essential for people with sickle cell anemia. Online forums, counseling services, and patient support groups are a few examples of these networks. Programs for financial aid and educational materials that are easily accessible may also help create a more encouraging atmosphere. The goal of these networks and services is to lessen the practical and emotional difficulties that patients and their families encounter.

## Coping Techniques For Families And Patients:

Managing social, emotional, and physical obstacles is a part of having sickle cell anemia. Creating healthy coping mechanisms is crucial for patients and their families alike. This might include developing resilience, getting mental health care, and using stress management strategies. Their quality of life may be much improved by fostering open communication within the family and giving them the resources they need to deal with the uncertainty brought on by the illness.

A more thorough and patient-centered approach to treating sickle cell anemia may be developed by incorporating these ideas into the general strategy. In addition to ensuring that those impacted by the illness get quality medical treatment, this also guarantees that they will gain from a community that is understanding, enlightened, and supportive.

# CHAPTER EIGHT

## Views From Around The World On Sickle Cell Anemia

### Review Of Sickle Cell Anemia:

A hereditary condition known as sickle cell anemia (SCA) is characterized by aberrant hemoglobin, which causes red blood cells to become deformed and resemble sickles. It is a global health issue that affects millions of people globally.

Examining the frequency of sickle cell anemia, differences in treatment accessibility, and international cooperation are necessary to comprehend viewpoints on the disease from a global perspective.

## Global Prevalence:

SCA is a common condition in many parts of the world, while it is more common in other places. The illness is more common in Sub-Saharan Africa, the Middle East, some regions of India, and several Mediterranean nations. Due to historical variables like malaria resistance, the frequency of the sickle cell gene is greater in certain places. The fact that migratory patterns have also resulted in pockets of SCA prevalence in other regions of the globe highlights the disease's worldwide reach.

Within groups, the frequency of SCA varies as well; those of African, Mediterranean, Middle Eastern, and Indian heritage seem to have greater rates. The disease's genetic component plays a role in its spread, highlighting the need to take genetic variation into account when assessing the disease's worldwide effect.

## Inequalities In Treatment Access:

Even with technological and scientific advancements in medicine, there are still large gaps in the therapeutic options available to people with SCA. These differences show themselves in a number of ways, including social, economic, and geographic aspects.

Comprehensive treatment for SCA is comparatively easier to get in many high-income nations since these nations have well-established healthcare infrastructures and specialized medical facilities. However, access to quality healthcare treatments may be restricted in low- and middle-income nations, especially in areas where SCA is more prevalent. These discrepancies are exacerbated by a lack of understanding, financial difficulties, and inadequate resources for healthcare.

Treatment accessibility is also influenced by social determinants of health, such as poverty and educational attainment. Healthcare hurdles for individuals with SCA who live in disadvantaged groups may include prejudice, stigma, and a lack of understanding. A multifaceted strategy is needed to address these discrepancies, including enhancing the healthcare system, increasing public awareness, and putting legislation in place that supports fair access to care.

## International Partnerships And Projects:

A greater focus is being placed on international partnerships and activities to solve the problems related to SCA, given the disease's widespread effects. To improve outcomes for people with SCA, a number of governmental and non-governmental groups have joined together to exchange information, pool resources, and put ideas into action.

Research, the exchange of best practices in healthcare delivery, and the promotion of treatment accessibility policies are the main areas of emphasis for international cooperation. These programs provide comprehensive plans for treating and preventing SCA by using the knowledge of scientists, healthcare practitioners, and policymakers from throughout the globe.

Initiatives also often target societal variables that lead to differences in SCA results, reaching beyond the healthcare industry. Advocacy, community involvement, and educational activities are essential parts of these joint projects.

To sum up, comprehending the global viewpoints on sickle cell anemia entails acknowledging the disease's ubiquity around the globe, tackling inequalities in treatment accessibility, and promoting global partnerships and endeavors. Through a comprehensive and cooperative approach, the international community may strive to enhance the quality of life for those impacted by sickle cell disease (SCA).

# CHAPTER NINE

## Awareness And Involvement In The Community

In order to effectively treat and manage sickle cell anemia, community participation is essential because it promotes teamwork that goes beyond medical treatments. In order to provide a supportive atmosphere, this all-encompassing approach calls for community awareness-raising and active engagement.

### The Value Of Participation In The Community

Participation in the community is important for many reasons. First of all, it makes sure that people are fully informed about sickle cell anemia by facilitating the spread of correct information about the illness. By becoming involved, community people develop into advocates and promote a feeling of collective accountability for handling the disease's issues. Involving the community also helps afflicted people establish a support system, which fosters a feeling of community and lessens the isolation that sickle cell anemia sufferers often face.

## Increasing Conscience

A fundamental component of the streamlined solution method is increasing public knowledge. The community may be educated about the causes, symptoms, and possible therapies for sickle cell anemia via the implementation of educational projects, campaigns, and outreach programs. This helps with early diagnosis and lessens the stigma and misunderstandings associated with the illness. A greater understanding enables people to make knowledgeable choices about getting medical help, taking preventative action, or providing support to others who are impacted.

## Taking Care Of Misconceptions And Stigmas

Misconceptions and stigmas related to sickle cell anemia may pose significant obstacles to receiving the right care and assistance. Participating in the community provides a forum for refuting and challenging these beliefs. The community may contribute toward dispelling prejudices and advancing empathy by encouraging candid conversation and disseminating correct facts. It must be made clear that sickle cell anemia is a medical issue and not a reflection of an individual's behavior. Communities may improve the quality of life for those with sickle cell anemia by working together to provide an environment of acceptance and understanding.

To summarize, a simple solution approach to sickle cell anemia must include community participation and awareness. We can all help create a culture that is more understanding and supportive by integrating the community, removing stigmas, and providing correct information. In the end, this will improve the quality of life for those who have sickle cell anemia.

# Conclusion

## Key Insights Recap:

Several important discoveries have been made along the trip via the simple solution approach to sickle cell anemia. Priority should be given to comprehending the disease's genetic foundation. A mutation in the HBB gene, which results in the generation of aberrant hemoglobin, is the main cause of sickle cell anemia. Any tailored therapeutic intervention starts with this realization.

Understanding the complexity of sickle cell anemia is another important realization. It impacts not only the red blood cells but also sets off a series of actions that affect the body's systems and organs. This complete knowledge is essential for creating all-encompassing treatment plans that take care of the disease's symptoms as well as its underlying causes.

Morcover, it is impossible to exaggerate the significance of an early diagnosis. For those with sickle cell anemia, early identification enables prompt intervention and therapy, reducing complications and enhancing overall quality of life. This highlights the need for greater awareness, frequent tests, and easily accessible medical services.

## The Path Ahead:

The fight against sickle cell anemia has both opportunities and difficulties ahead of us.

The prospect of rectifying the genetic mutation causing the illness is significant because of advancements in genetic therapy, which include gene editing tools like CRISPR-Cas9. However, the difficulties in putting these innovative ideas into practice are highlighted by safety concerns, ethical issues, and the need for thorough clinical studies.

Furthermore, it is essential to make a concentrated effort in initiatives for education and awareness. By debunking falsehoods, lowering stigma, and advocating genetic counseling, we may enable people and communities to make informed choices about family planning, which will eventually lower the disease's prevalence.

# Prospects And Obstacles:

Notwithstanding the difficulties, there is optimism for a day when sickle cell anemia will be adequately treated and, preferably, completely eliminated. To get past the obstacles on this path, cooperation between academics, medical experts, legislators, and impacted communities is crucial. A more fair and successful strategy for treating sickle cell anemia may be made possible by developments in customized medicine and a focus on addressing the socioeconomic variables that contribute to health inequities.

Significant barriers, nevertheless, include things like scarce resources, uneven access to healthcare, and the need for international collaboration. To overcome these obstacles, one must be dedicated to promoting diversity, advocating for changes in policies, and making investments in healthcare infrastructure and research.

In summary, a thorough grasp of the genetic, medical, and social elements of sickle cell anemia is essential to the simple solution approach to the condition. We can work toward a future where the effects of sickle cell anemia are reduced and those who are affected can lead healthier, more fulfilling lives by building on important discoveries, navigating the path ahead with a combination of cutting-edge therapies and community engagement, and facing challenges with tenacity and collaboration.

# THE END